A Small Guide
To Building Bigger Arms

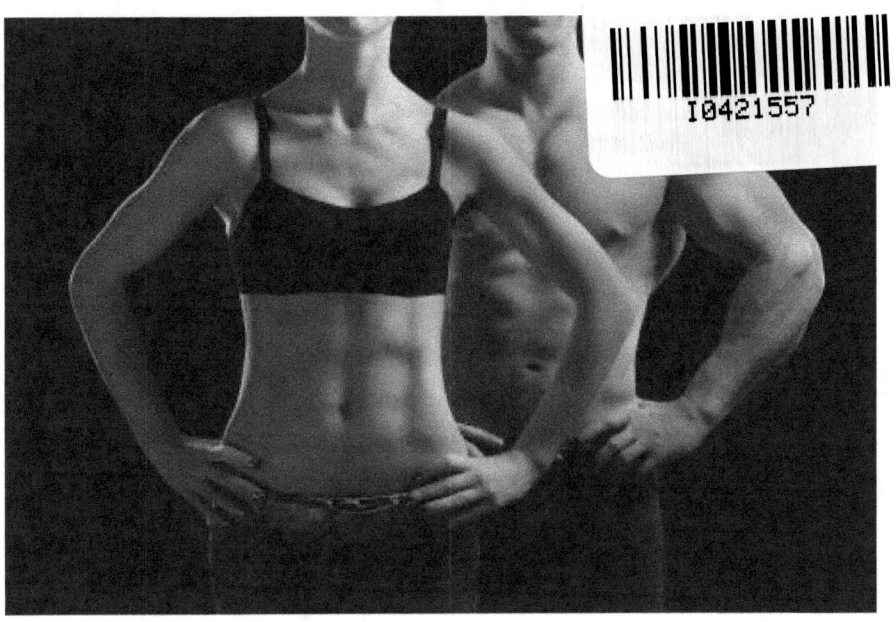

I0421557

Health Learning Series

M. Usman

Mendon Cottage Books

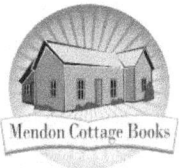

JD-Biz Publishing

All Rights Reserved.

Disclaimer

The information is this book is provided for informational purposes only. It is not intended to be used and medical advice or a substitute for proper medical treatment by a qualified health care provider. The information is believed to be accurate as presented based on research by the author.

The contents have not been evaluated by the U.S. Food and Drug Administration or any other Government or Health Organization and the contents in this book are not to be used to treat cure or prevent disease.

The author or publisher is not responsible for the use or safety of any diet, procedure, or treatment mentioned in this book. The author or publisher is not responsible for errors or omissions that may exist.

Warning

The Book is for informational purposes only and before taking on any diet, treatment, or medical procedure, it is recommended to consult with your primary health care provider.

Our books are available at

1. Amazon.com
2. Barnes and Noble
3. Itunes
4. Kobo
5. Smashwords
6. Google Play Books

Table of Contents

Preface

When trying to determine how muscular one is, the arms are usually the first indicator. While not everyone might be able to grow their arms easily, just a little muscle goes a long way in giving you pride.

Building your arms will not only make them grow in size, but they will also become stronger. Activities that used to make you sweat will start feeling like a piece of cake. As if that's not enough, big arms will get you compliments from both men and women.

But to achieve that, you will need to listen to the right advice. Exercise alone will not do it. If you are serious about getting big arms, read this book now, as it has everything you must know to get the arms you dream of.

Enjoy the reading.

Chapter # 1: The Role of Nutrition in Bodybuilding

When newbies talk of building muscles, they only focus on workouts. But, the truth is that getting the body you dream of needs a balance among a number of things and nutrition is one of them. In this chapter you will learn all about proper nutrition for bigger arms or any part of the body that you are trying to make muscular.

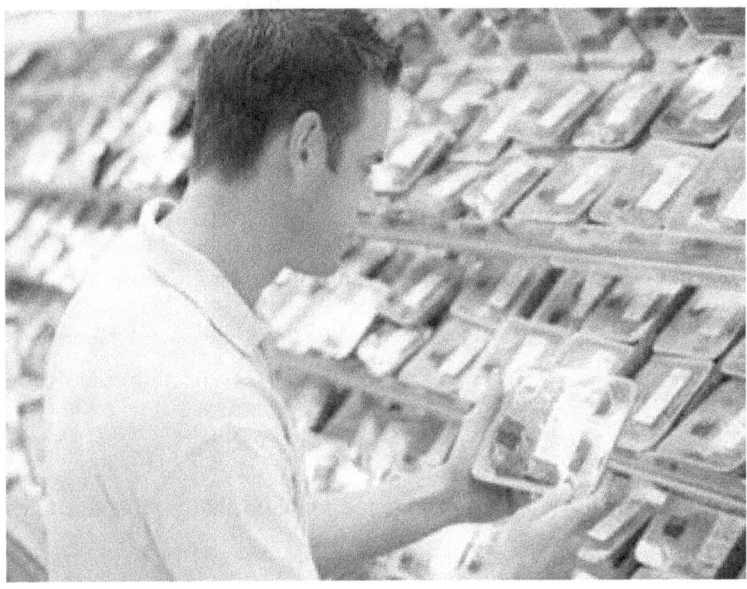

Benefits of Proper Nutrition

Eating the right foods is one of the cornerstones of bodybuilding. You can train as much as you want, but, if your diet is out of place, you will not see the results you deserve. Below are some of the reasons why the right food is important:

For energy – Food gives us the energy needed for survival every day. And when you are a bodybuilder, you will want to have even more energy than couch potatoes do. Otherwise, you will feel too exhausted to complete your workouts.

For growth – Food is also responsible for muscle growth. For bodybuilders, protein is the most important nutrient. However, that does not mean you should neglect other nutrients; they are all important for good health.

Manufacturing of hormones for muscle growth – Nutrients are also responsible in the production of hormones needed to have bigger muscles. For example, fats are used in the making of testosterone which is a hormone that promotes muscle growth.

How Often to Eat

Now that you understand why food is important for bigger arms, the next question is about the frequency of eating. Bodybuilders are encouraged to have 6 meals per day, rather than the traditional 3 or 4. Eating frequently will guarantee that you have a constant supply of energy all the time. Furthermore, the body will be getting all the necessary nutrients needed for muscle growth.

Before you get into a workout, it is recommended that you have some kind of a small meal. This must be consumed 1 or 2 hrs before the workout. Additionally, you should have a protein shake 20 minutes before the workout. If this is not done, you body may start breaking cells for energy, which is counterproductive.

How Much Should You Eat

Saying you need a lot of energy when bodybuilding does not give you a right to eat as much as you can. You still need to watch your portion sizes, since you will be eating frequently, your meals should be small.

What Should You Eat

Eating healthy food is everywhere these days and bodybuilding is not an exception. If you are consuming food that has no value, do not expect to see any change in your arms. As a matter of fact, do not be surprised if you begin gaining fat instead of muscle. So, what should you eat?

Proteins – This nutrient is important in every bodybuilder's diet. In fact, it is the number one nutrient to get enough of if you are building muscles. Protein is responsible for building new cells, repairing damaged muscles, and other functions. Best sources include eggs, whey protein, lean meats, beans, etc.

Fats – It's not all fat that is bad, as there is a type you need for a healthy life. Good fats come from foods like avocados, olive oil, salmon, sardines, nuts, etc. Saturated and Trans fats are not healthy and so must be avoided. However, saturated fat is used in the making of testosterone, so a little of it will not kill you.

Carbohydrates – This nutrient provides your cells with the energy you need to do your workouts and stay alive. But, make it a point to only consume healthy carbs. These include oatmeal, whole wheat bread, potatoes, brown rice, whole grain corn, etc. Refined carbohydrates are bad and must be limited in your diet.

Vitamins and Minerals – Although these are needed in small quantities, they are important nonetheless. So, include colorful fruits and vegetables on your plate.

Supplements – In recent years, there has been an increase in the number of people using bodybuilding supplements. Since they work, you can incorporate these in your diet as well. Just make sure you do not become too dependent on supplements.

Water – Dehydration is crucial when you are trying to build muscles, since you lose a lot of water during workouts. So, drink at least eight 8-ounce glasses of water daily. If you are feeling thirsty frequently, it means you are not drinking enough.

Food is important when you are building muscles. However, it's not all food that will give you bigger muscles, so you will need to eat clean. Food that has undergone heavy processing should not find its way into your stomach often.

Chapter # 2: How Long Should You Train

You may be terrified to learn that there are bodybuilders who stay in the gym for 2 hours or more working on a single muscle. Thankfully, it is not everyone who needs to train like that. In this chapter, I will discuss all about this subject.

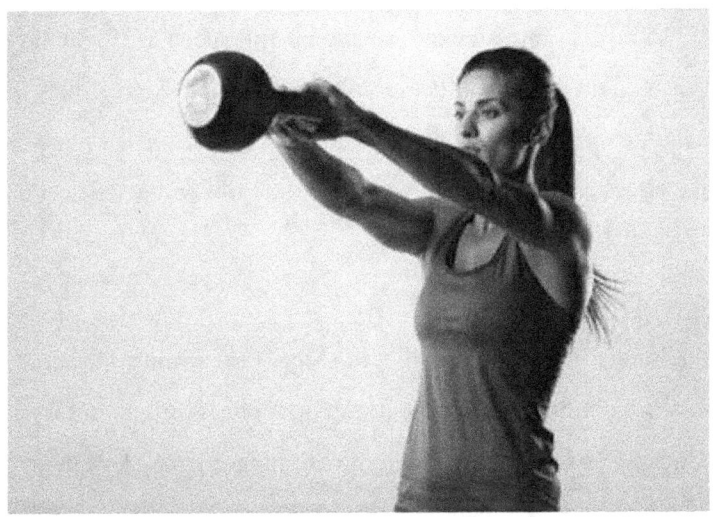

Things to Consider When Determining How Long to Train

If we were made the same way, it would be simple to tell anyone how long they should train. But the painful truth is that we are different. And it's our differences that make it necessary to consider a few things before determining how long you should exercise. With the same training frequency and workouts, people will have different results. That is enough proof that we are not equal.

Fitness Level

Sickness, age, gender, and other factors contribute to strength. Before you can decide how long you should be training, take time to think if you are capable of achieving the goal you have set. For example, if you are over the age of 50, saying you will run 5 miles, if you have never managed to finish a mile, is absurd. So be honest with yourself. You can seek help from someone who is experienced to help you here.

Experience

It is dumb to just get into an exercise and hit full speed as if you have been at it for years. You will likely get an injury in the end. Start slowly and build your strength over time. Not only will you teach your muscles how to handle the stress associated with workouts, but you will also learn proper form.

Training Duration

In life, the longer you do something, the bigger the results. However, when it comes to bodybuilding, that rule does not apply. Working out for longer periods does not mean you will end up with bigger arms. As a matter of fact, you will be lucky to see much progress.

Exercising for too long leads to overtraining, something that goes against every rule of bodybuilding. Muscles only grow when given time to recover. So, sleep for 6–8 hours daily. Additionally, avoid training every day, as that will leave your muscles stressed all the time.

The rule is that if your workouts are very intense, you do not need to do them for too long. Just 45 minutes is all you need. And, since we are just focusing on building arms here, 3 days per week might be all you need to see results.

When Will You See Results

If you are doing everything right, you should start feeling the fruits of your labor in just a few weeks. Specifically, it takes 4 to 8 weeks for muscles to start growing. But, you will also notice that workouts will become easier with time. That is your green light that things are turning out the way they should be.

If you are not seeing results, it means there are some important things you are missing and these must be rectified right away.

Chapter # 3: Warming Up

Many beginners usually skip warming up and simply jump into action. However, that is a recipe for disaster when it comes to bodybuilding. Since we sit a lot, our muscles need to be prepared for whatever exercise we plan on doing.

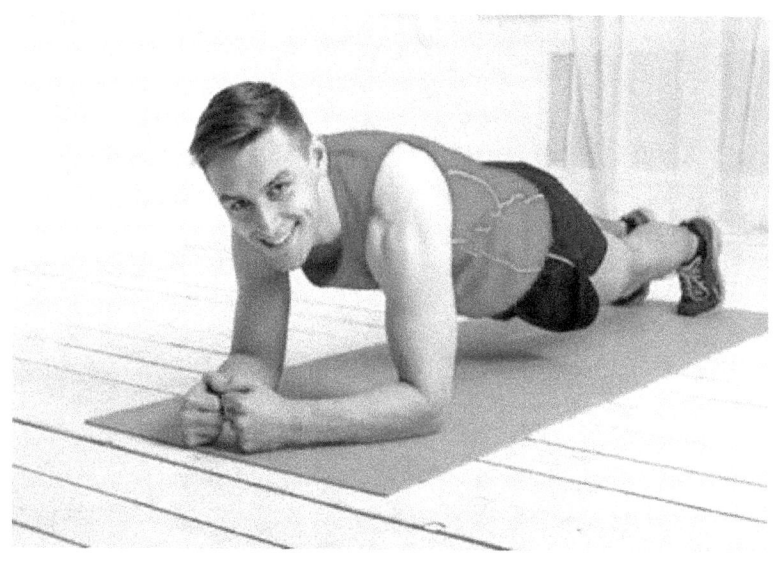

And when it's the arms in question, the benefits of warming up cannot be overemphasized. Being one of the most used parts of the body, you surely would not want to end up with an injured arm.

The Benefits of Warming Up
Below are some of the benefits of a proper warm-up:

Increases muscle temperature – Warming up increases muscle temperature, which in turn reduces the risk of injury, as heated muscles contract easily and quickly.

Increases blood flow – A warm-up increases your heart rate, which results in more blood rushing through your veins. This boosts oxygen levels directed to your cells, giving you more energy.

Makes the joints flexible – The amount of synovial fluid being released is raised after a warm-up. This fluid is responsible for lubricating your joints for maximum flexibility.

Prepares you psychologically – This is probably the most undervalued benefit of warming up. Achieving something requires not only your physical state, but your mental willingness, as well. If your mind is not into it, you will have a hard time fulfilling your dreams.

How to Warm-Up for Arm Workouts
Regardless of what kind of workout you are planning on doing, your warm-up does not need to feel like a main workout. As long as the arms are heated and you have got the heart pumping, your mission has been achieved. So, do not feel ashamed if you think your warm-up is a joke.

Run

Despite the fact that we are focusing on the arms here, it's your whole body that will be involved in the workout. Running is a better way to get every part of the body ready for whatever workout is to follow. So run for 3 or 4 minutes.

Arm Circles

This little exercise is meant to prepare the arms and shoulders. Start by standing with your feet about shoulder-width apart. Spread your arms to the sides so that you are making a T with your body. Once in position, start making circles with your arms. Do this for 10 reps. Remember to also do it in reverse.

Do a Mini Version of Your Main Workout

Doing a mini version of your main workout is also a great way to get your arms ready. So if you know you will be lifting weights, getting down with a lighter weight will be very effective in getting your body ready.

Just as I said previously, there is no need to make a warm-up feel like the main exercise. You will only get yourself exhausted. Depending on your fitness level and type of workout you plan on doing, you should set 5 to 10 minutes for warm-ups. For total flexibility, however, I would recommend that you do it for 10 minutes.

Chapter # 4: Exercises for Shoulders

Big, wide, and strong shoulders make a man. That's something that has been programmed into our minds. And no matter how big you are, if you shoulders look like they belong on a deer, do not expect to wow anyone with your physique.

Unfortunately, many think of big arms as having impressive triceps and biceps; shoulders are an afterthought. But if you are serious about getting gigantic arms, do not neglect your shoulders.

Formation of the Shoulders

Know that you know the importance of big shoulders you might be tempted to jump into action. However, that will be a mistake. You first need to understand how your shoulders are made.

Contrary to what many think, each shoulder is made up of three muscles called deltoids. These are named as the anterior deltoid, medial deltoid, and posterior deltoid.

Of the three, the anterior deltoid is the one that usually gets involved in workouts; for example, when you are doing chest workouts. But since you will want impressive shoulders in general, all three deltoids must be engaged in your workouts. Otherwise, you will look funny in the end.

Best Exercises for Massive Shoulders

There are a lot of exercises meant to result in titanic like shoulders. However, results differ depending on the type of workouts you are focusing on. Other exercises will give you better results and at a faster rate. Below are some of the most highly rated shoulder exercises.

1. The Military Press

The military press is certainly one of the best shoulder exercises you can do. The best part is that this workout hits all three deltoids, setting you up for success. Additionally, there is minimal risk of injury with the military press (only those who are reckless should expect an injury).

The military press can be done in two ways: while seated or standing. The seated version is easier making it a good option for those who are just getting started. If you are looking for faster results, the standing military press might be the way to go.

To start out, do 3 sets with 8–12 reps, depending on your fitness level.

2. Side/Front/Rear Delt Raise

These are other shoulder workouts that involve all the three deltoids. If you have never done a delt raise before, start with lighter weights. You will have to do 3 sets of the side delt raise, 3 sets of the front delt raise and 3 sets of the rear delt raise. In each set, do 8–12 reps.

3. Handstand Pushup

No equipment? Not a problem! Your own body is the greatest equipment you can ever need. With the handstand pushup, you will build strong and massive shoulders. Making it even better is the fact that all three muscles that make up the shoulders are involved.

However, this workout takes some time to perfect. For beginners, learn to get into a handstand pushup position first and hold it for a minute. Once you achieve that, you will be ready to start doing the actual pushup.

Chapter # 5: Exercises for Bigger Triceps

Many are not aware of the fact that the triceps make up about 2/3 of the upper arm. So, it is not surprising to see that the majority of people trying to build bigger arms focus on the wrong exercises. Not only does that waste valuable time, but it's also a surefire way to get discouraged, as you will not see the results you want.

With enormous triceps, it will be easy for anyone to notice that you have stupendous arms. Adding to that, working your triceps will improve your overall strength, as they are the muscles that make up a good proportion of your upper arms. Furthermore, studies have showed that strong triceps improve your performance in other exercises.

Formation of the Triceps

Just like with the shoulders, many mistakenly think that triceps are made up of one group of muscle. But actually, it is three groups of muscles. These are the lateral head, medial head, and long head. All three must be involved in your workouts for overall huge triceps.

Exercises

There are a range of exercises targeting the triceps. In this chapter, I have included only the best. In choosing these exercises, efficiency and effectiveness were the determinants. In essence, that means the workouts below involve all three major muscles of the triceps at once and still manages to give you great results.

1. Triceps Dips

If you are serious about increasing the size of your triceps, dips must be on your menu. This workout is among the best that hits all three triceps muscles at once.

If you do not have the right equipment, there is no need to worry. Triceps dips have many variations, with some not requiring any kind of special equipment. For starters, 3 sets with 10 – 12 reps will do.

2. Closed-Grip Bench Press

This is another workout that targets all three major muscles, guaranteeing that you will get definition in your triceps. At the same time, the chest is also involved to some extent. As with the other exercises, 3 sets of 8–10 reps, should get you started. However, make it a point to learn the proper technique of doing this workout.

3. Overhead Dumbbell Extension

Although the emphasis is on the long head, the other 2 muscles also get some level of stimulation. Again, proper technique is important with this exercise. If done wrong, there is always the risk of injury.

4. Dumbbell Kickbacks

This is my favorite exercise for massive triceps. It too works all three muscles. However, because of its nature, you will need to use lighter weights when you are just beginning. Otherwise, you will add stress to your shoulders which might result in injury down the road.

Chapter # 6: Exercises for Biceps

The biceps get more attention than they deserve. Justifying my argument is the fact that this muscle group only makes up about 1/3 of the upper arm. Nonetheless, it is important to take time working on it. As a matter of fact, it is what people mainly use to measure your muscularity.

Just make it a point to not treat the biceps as your only muscles. Rather, regard them as a small part of your overall physique.

Formation of the Biceps

Similar to the shoulders and the triceps, the biceps are also a group of three muscles. These are the biceps brachii, coracobrachialis, and brachialis. Together, these make up just 1/3 of the upper arm.

Exercises to Perform

If you have ever done any bodybuilding exercises before, chances are that you already did some biceps workouts. Here are some of the best workouts that will make you stand out when flexing.

1. Barbell Biceps Curls

Barbell biceps curls must be on your list, because they are very effective. This workout gives your biceps enough resistance needed for growth. Even better, it is hard to cheat when doing a biceps curl.

I cannot overemphasize the importance of going slowly if you are just starting out. Trying to make quick gains will force you to adopt bad habits that will be difficult to get rid of down the road.

2. Concentration Curls

I love this exercise for one reason; you do it while sitting down. So there is a reduction in movement making it possible for you to just focus on the biceps. As always, do 3 sets of 8 reps for a start. If you notice that the exercise is getting easier, increase the intensity.

3. Standing Biceps Cable Curls

Although there is movement in this workout, you will still be able to grow your biceps and make them stronger. If you can't go to a gym for this exercise, any band that gives your biceps enough resistance should do.

4. Hammer Curl

This workout is also meant to give you bigger and powerful biceps. Making it even better, your forearms will also be involved.

5. Chin Ups

When done right, this is one of the best biceps exercises you can ever do. It gives the biceps resistance, as they need to pull your body up until your chin is level with the bar. Apart from building size, chin-ups are also great for building strength. Just make sure you are not cheating and your body is straight as you do this.

Chapter # 7: Avoiding the Plateau

You might think that doing all the exercises above will automatically lead to bigger arms, but that is not always the case with a lot of people.

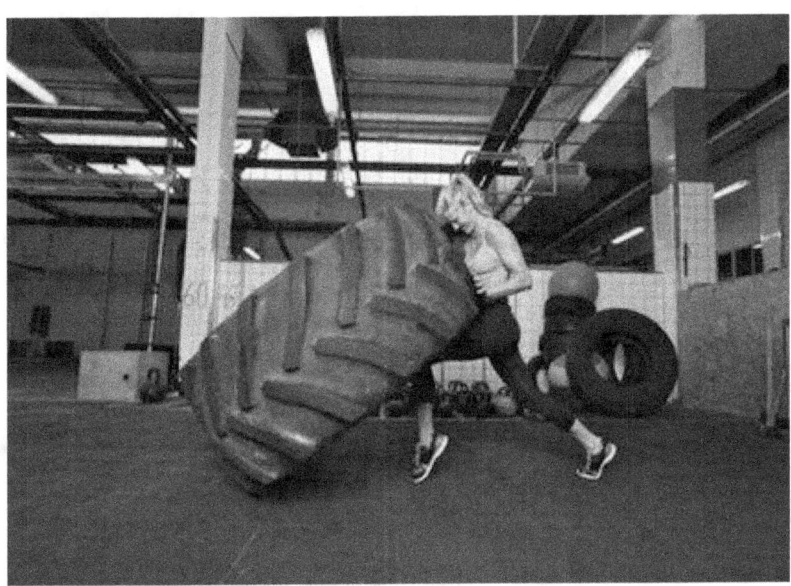

Your body can adapt to your workouts thereby hurting your progress.

How the Body Adapts

When we exercise, we place a lot of stress on the muscles. That is what results in growth. But with time, the muscles will figure out ways of making the workouts easier.

When that happens, you will notice that your muscle size is not growing as fast as when you had just started. Additionally, you will also realize that the exercises have become easier. This is called a plateau. If nothing changes, forget about the possibility of looking like Arnold Schwarzenegger.

Fortunately, there are a number of ways you can use to get off from this plateau or stop it from happening in the first place. By far, variety is the best solution for plateaus. Depending on your preferences, below are some of the solutions:

1. Change Sets

As you saw in this book, most of the workouts emphasized doing 3 sets with 8–10 reps. However, with time, your muscles will adapt to that kind of a setup.

So, after every 3 or 4 weeks, change how your workout is composed. Instead of going for 3 sets with 10 reps, try 10 sets with 3 reps. That will surprise your muscles and they will be stressed, giving you assurance that they will keep on growing.

2. Change Exercises

This is also among the best ways to avoid setting yourself up for a plateau. Have a list of exercises for each part of your body, and after 2 or 3 weeks, change to another exercise. For example, if you have been doing dumbbell barbell curls for 2 weeks, start doing chin ups.

Having a notebook to record your exercises will be beneficial in planning.

3. Increase/Decrease Training Time

Changing the amount of time devoted to each workout can also work in your favor. If your workouts have been lasting for an hour, you might try going for 45 minutes while increasing intensity.

5. Increase Frequency

If you have been working out 3 times a week, you can increase the rate to 4 or 5 times. That will put more stress on your muscles. However, reduce the intensity of your workouts so that the body has enough time to recover.

These tips are not only valid for those building bigger arms. You can apply the same techniques when trying to build any muscle in the body.

Chapter # 8: Introduction to Injuries

Not only are big arms impressive to look at, but they also boost your confidence. However, those benefits come at a cost in the form of an injury. You can do your best to avoid being injured, but sometimes, you may be at the wrong place at the wrong time.

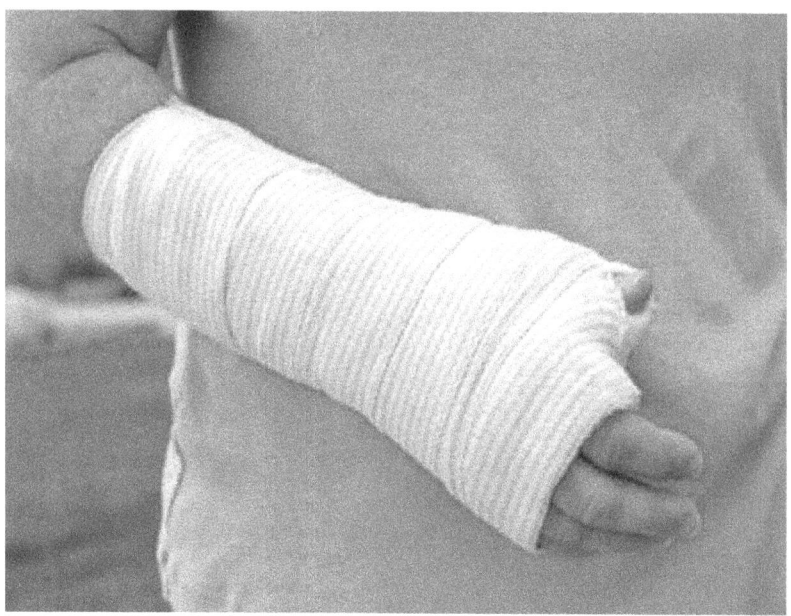

So it is crucial that we address this important issue of injuries.

Usually, injuries in the arms have to do with the shoulders. But this does not mean the possibility of pulling any muscle in the arms is zero.

Types of Injuries
There are two types of injuries. Let's discuss them below:

1. Acute Injuries

Acute means something that just happens rapidly. In the same sense, acute injuries occur swiftly. An example would be falling and hurting any part of your arm. You will feel pain right away signifying that there has been damage. In some situations, you may also experience swelling as well as bleeding.

2. Chronic Injuries

This is the opposite of acute, as these are injuries that develop slowly until they become full-blown injuries capable of restricting you from performing. Usually, this is a result of not paying attention to your body's cues that you may have an injury.

Causes of Arm Injuries

If you do everything right, the possibility of having an arm injury is very low. However, we usually ignore the basics raising the risk of hurting ourselves. Below are some of the causes of injuries:

1. Inadequate warm-up – Many beginners like to skip or rush through the warm-up. This is a clear sign of someone who missed a class on the importance of warming up properly. Due to our sedentary lifestyles, our muscles are not always active. And to start stressing them while they are cold and stiff is the best way to nurture disaster.

2. Incorrect Technique – With heavy weights, there is always the risk of cheating in order to pull off the exercise. However, this might introduce bad habits that will result in muscles moving in ways they are not supposed to.

3. Going beyond capabilities – The fact that we are all human does not mean our fitness levels are also the same. If someone younger than you is lifting more than you can, give them respect. But do not attempt to outshine them. You are not yet ready to go head to head with someone like that. It takes time to build strength, so do not be ashamed of taking it slowly.

4. Overuse – It was stated earlier in the book, but it deserves a second mention here: your body needs to recover from your workouts. Without enough resting time, you will likely develop chronic injuries, as muscles will be stressed all the time.

5. Restrictive Clothes – Wearing the right clothes is also important when it comes to building arms. If your clothes do not give you freedom to move, you will end up injured. At the same time, if they are saggy and they get in your way, expect the worst as well.

Chapter # 9: Treatment and Prevention of Injuries

With an injury, it will be impossible to achieve your dreams. And if the injury persists, it might as well be the end of the road.

Treating injuries is not difficult, as long as you understand the nature of your injury. If it is not so severe, you can treat it yourself at home.

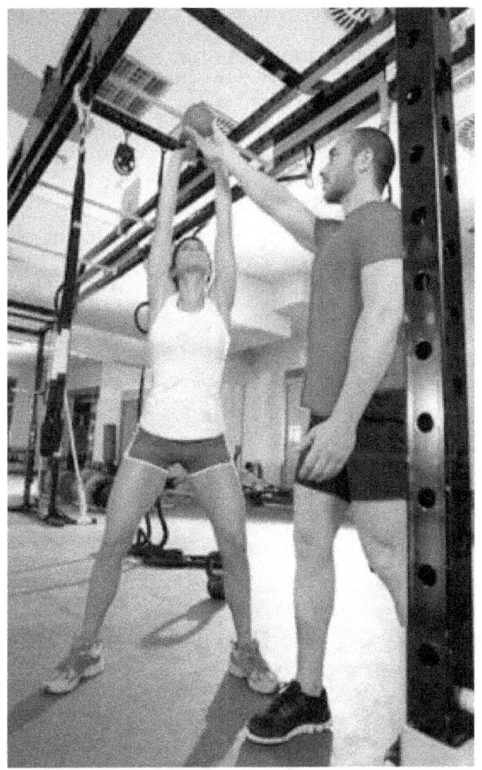

If your injury is acute and it is restricting movement or it is painful, you should use the RICE technique. This method, however, is only valuable in the first 48–72 hours of injury.

Rest – The "R" means rest. Since your body will start the healing process soon after the injury, you should make it a point to avoid further damage. If you had scheduled a workout, postpone it or choose other exercises that do not make use of the injured part.

Ice – The "I" is for ice. 15 minutes after the injury, apply ice to the wounded part, as it reduces blood flow, thereby lessening pain and inflammation. However, remove the ice if your skin starts feeling numb and only apply again when your body temperature returns to normal.

Compression – "C" stands for compression. Keeping the wounded part compressed is also a great way to reduce pain and inflammation. The best way to achieve this is by using a bandage.

Elevation – The "E" is for elevation. With regard to the laws of gravity, you can keep blood away from the wounded part by raising your arm above the heart.

After the 72 hours, strive to prevent further damage to your arm. You should only start using it after it has fully recovered. The severity of your injury will determine how long it will take before you can get back to your arm building exercises.

Furthermore, you are encouraged to keep doing exercises that do not involve the injured part. Since we are building arms in this book, walking, jogging and other similar exercises will be a good option. By the time you recover, you will still be in good shape.

If your injury is serious or if your condition does not improve after a couple of days, it is recommended that you see a doctor.

Preventing Injuries

The best treatment to any injury is to keep it from happening in the first place. By following a number of ways, you will realize how easy that is.

Firstly, you must know the risk factors. For example, using the wrong equipment or being too close to someone can all result in injuries. Once you know the risk factors, come up with ways to address them.

Here are additional things to keep in mind:

Warm Up – The importance of warming up cannot be overemphasized. In chapter three, I gave you everything needed to properly warm up your arms.

Use the correct technique – Simply reading about how to do a certain workout is not the best way to learn it. I would recommend that you work with a trained coach if you are just starting out. Learning how your body should move is crucial in preventing injuries.

Listen to your body – The saying "no pain no gain" is what misleads many. Pain is your body's system of telling you that something is amiss. If ignored, you will keep on abusing your muscles. By the time you will realize it, a chronic injury will be already on your door.

Know your fitness level – You should never force yourself to go beyond your capabilities. It takes time to build muscle endurance and strength. Think of it as taking a single step at a time. You are the only person you have to impress in the end.

Conclusion

Having gotten this far, I would first like to congratulate you. I am positive that the book gave you all the information you were looking for in order to get bigger arms.

Along with the exercises, remember to also put nutrition in the forefront. The exercises alone are not enough to give you the results you want. Additionally, learn how to do each exercise properly in order to reduce the risk of an injury. Getting enough sleep is also important, because it will give your muscles a chance to recover and keep on growing. If you do all these things, you will surely see your arms get bigger.

However, do not treat your arms as if they are your only body part. Take time to also workout the rest of your body, including your legs, chest, and back. Including all muscles in your workouts will make you look balanced. Furthermore, you should also include aerobic exercises at least once a week.

Good luck on your journey, and thank you for reading!

Author Bio

Muhammad Usman is a distinguished medical graduate of Allama Iqbal medical college (AIMC). He is a professional writer who has been in the field for more than 4 years. During this time he has produced 10,000+ articles, blogs, and eBooks on various niches related to diseases, health, fitness, nutrition, and well-being. He is a regular contributor to several journals related to medicine and surgery. He is the editor of several journals and newspapers.

Check out some of the other JD-Biz Publishing books

Gardening Series on Amazon

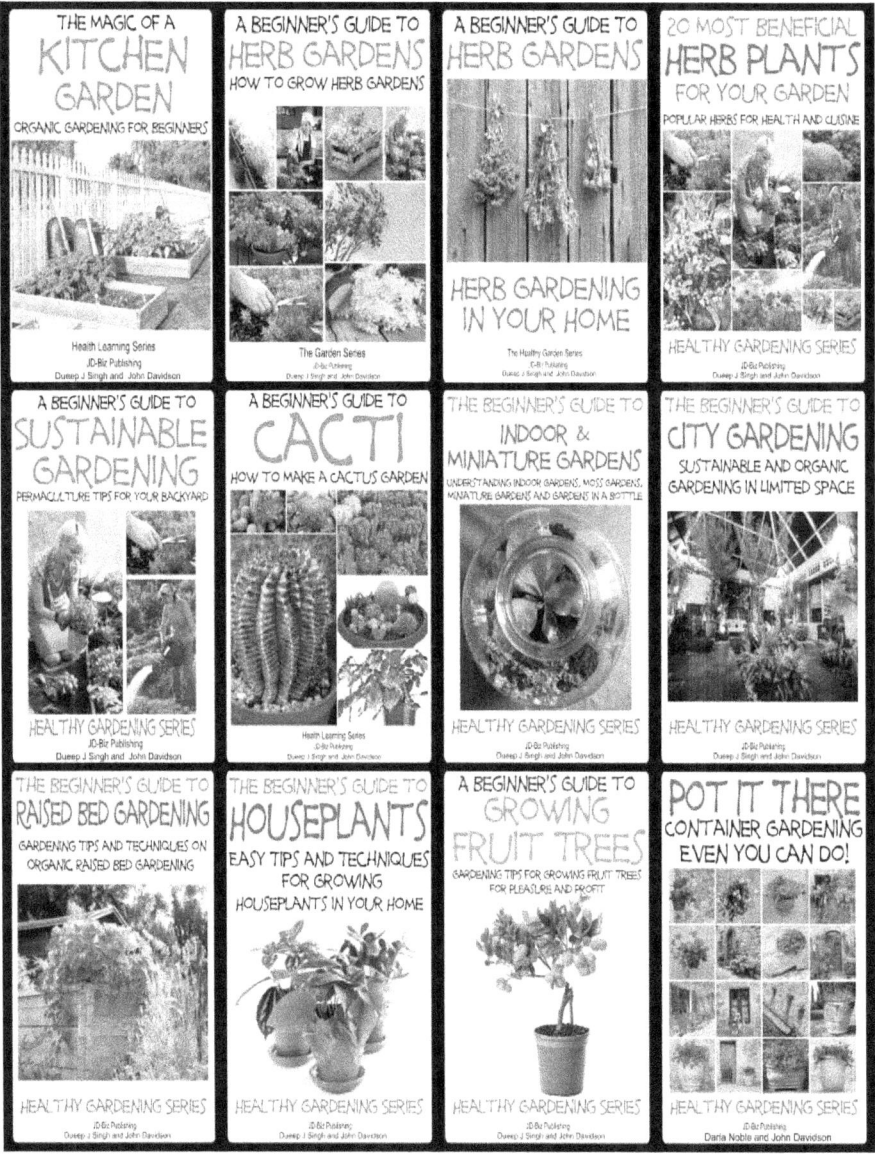

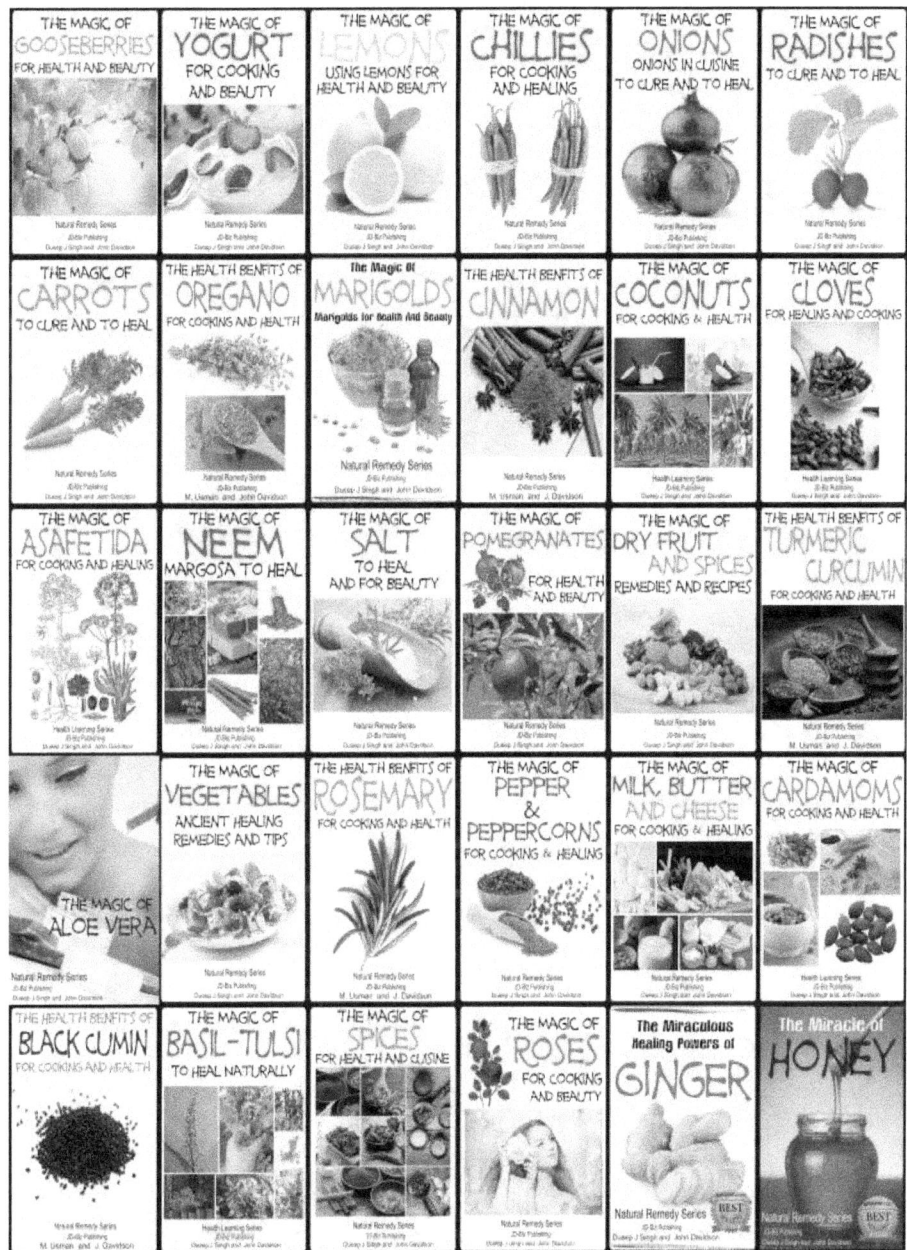

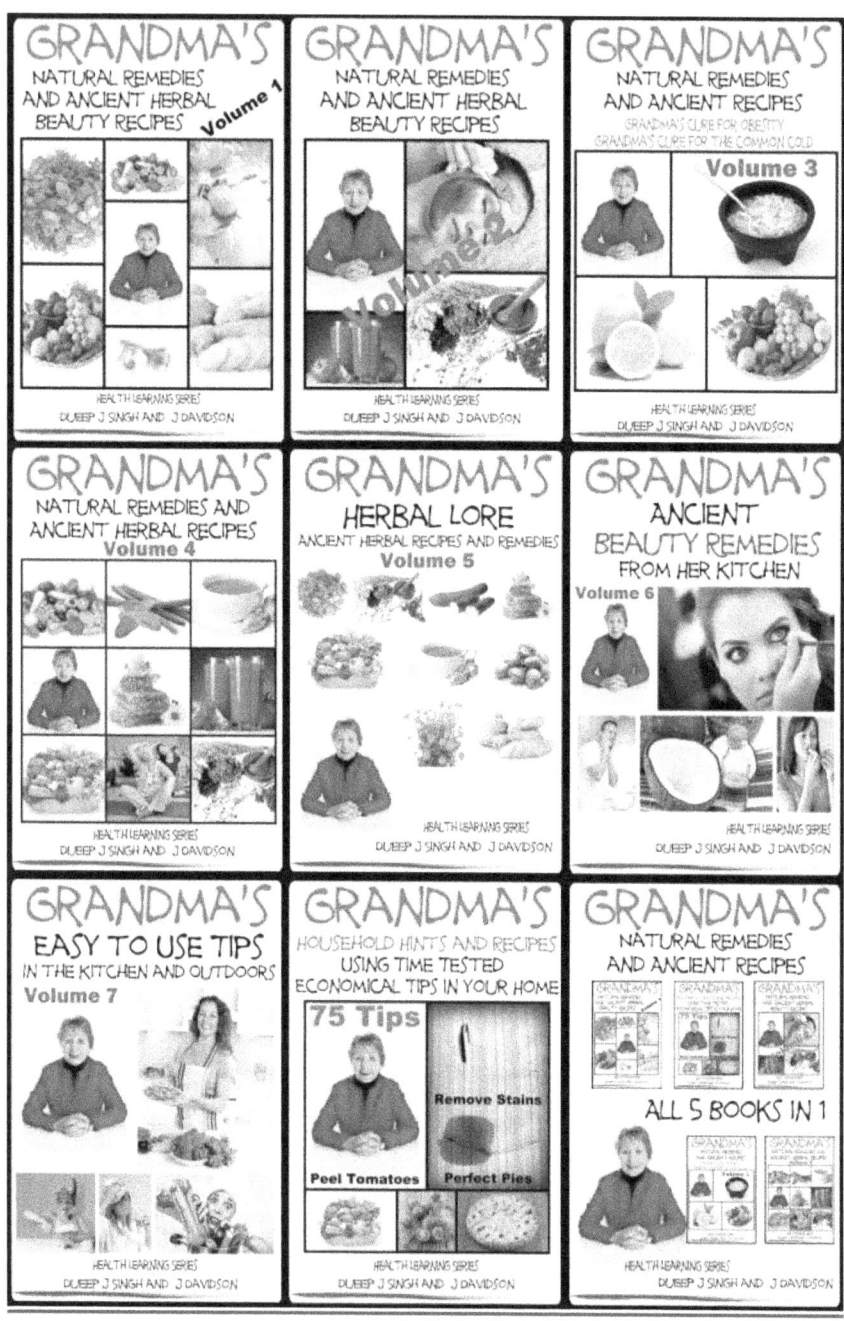

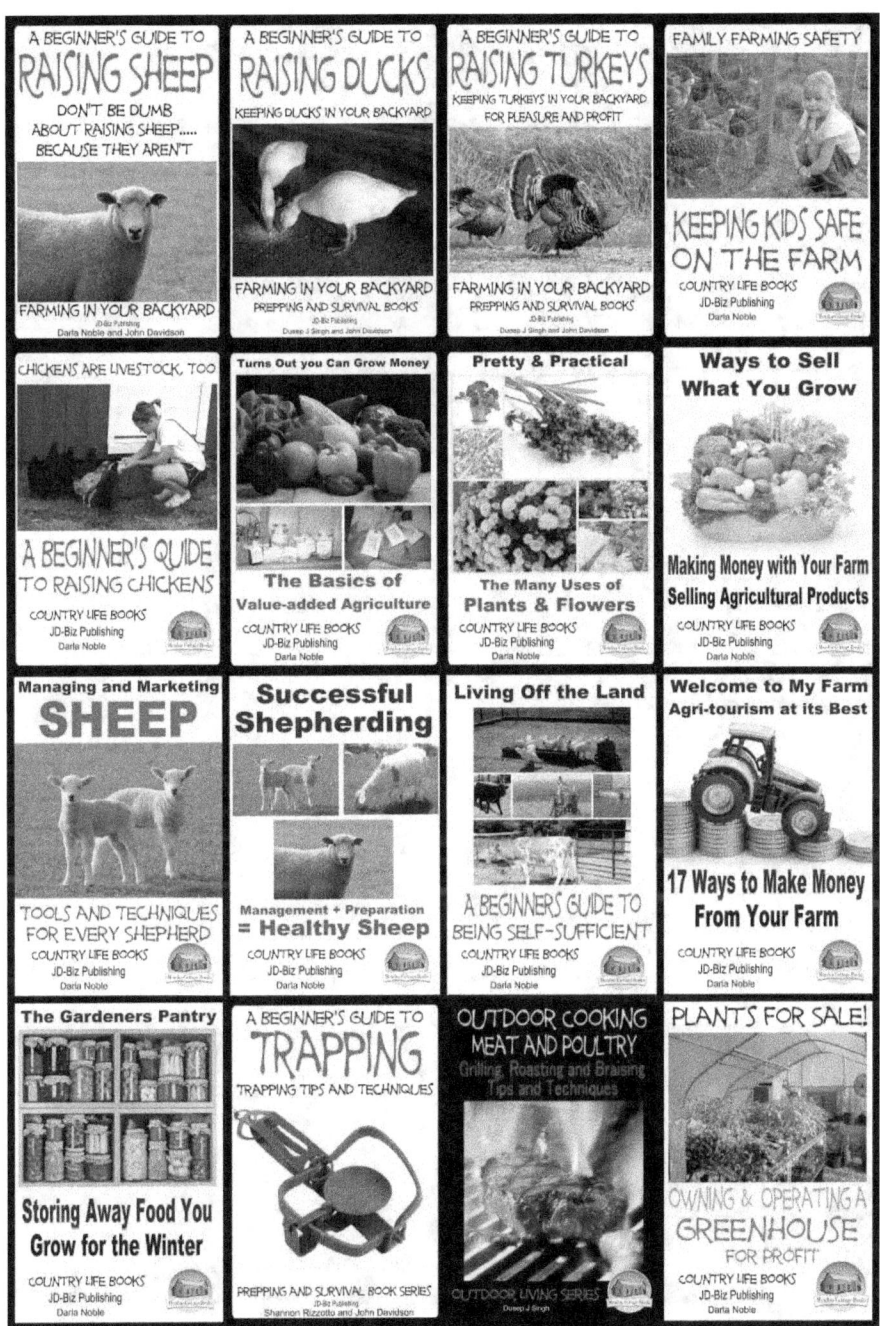

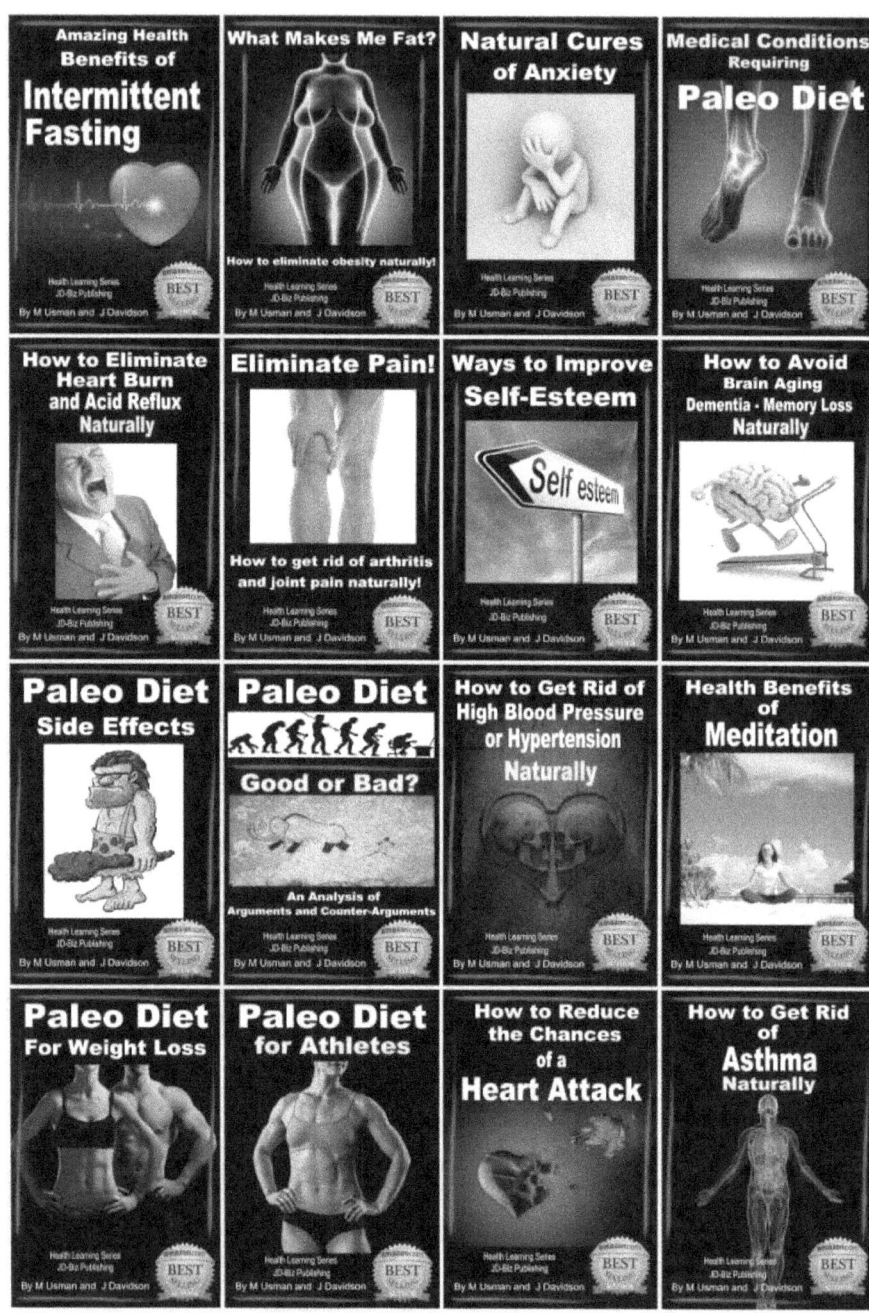

Amazing Animal Book Series

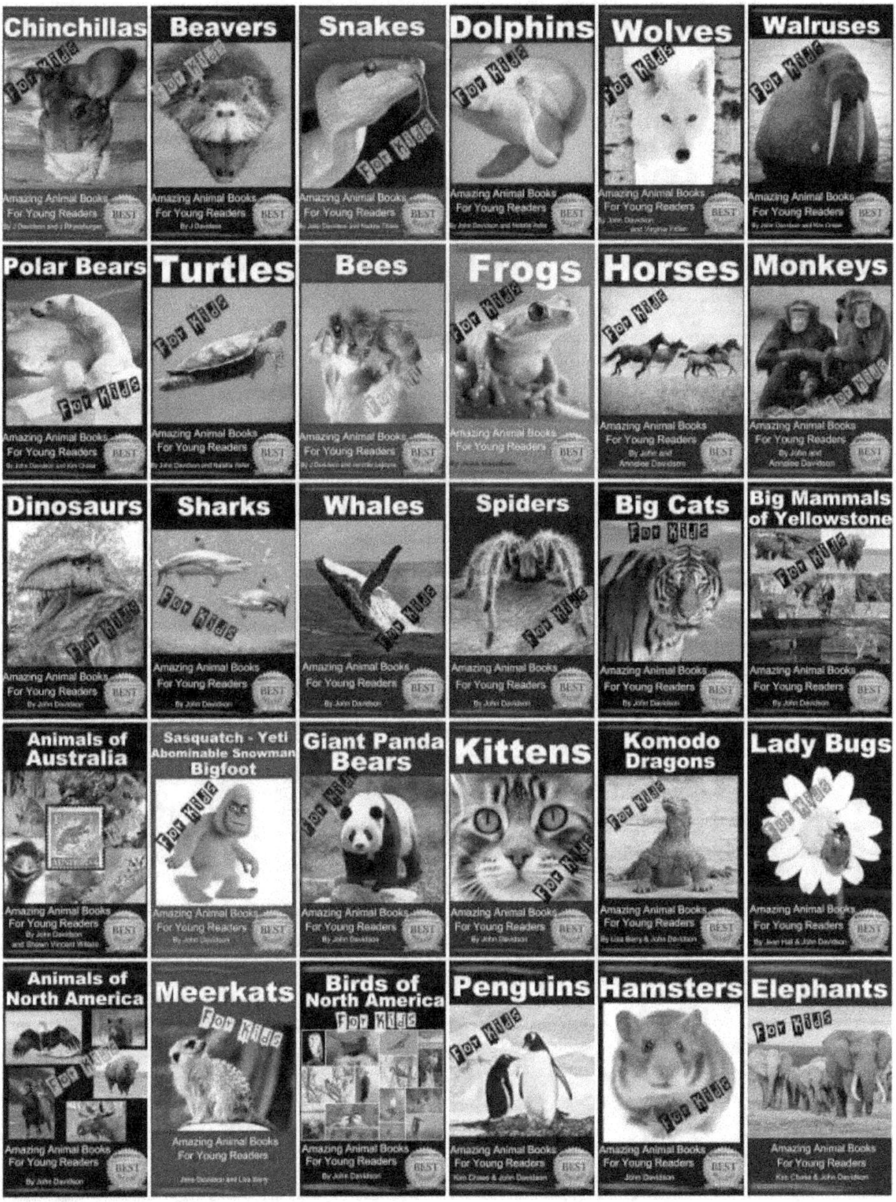

Learn To Draw Series

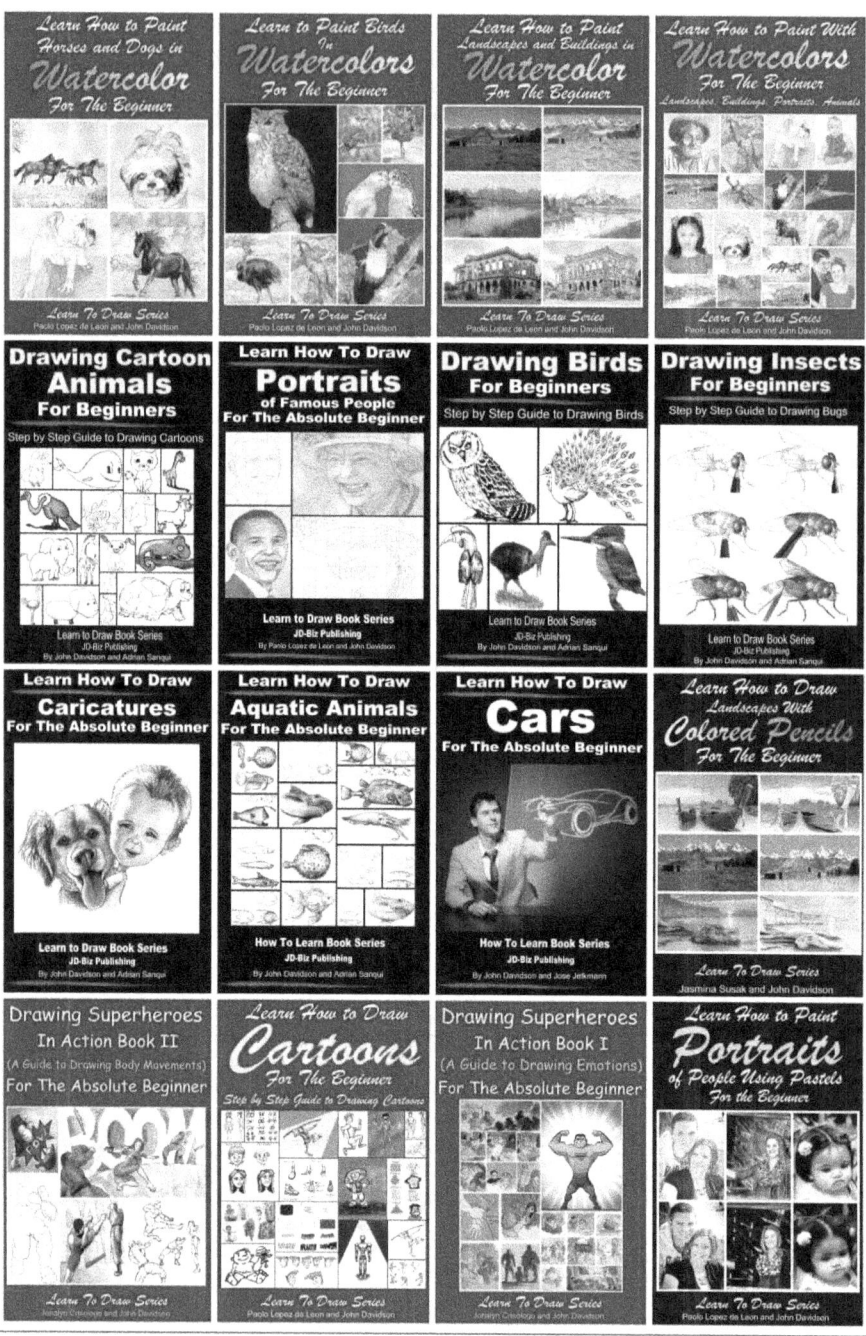

How to Build and Plan Books

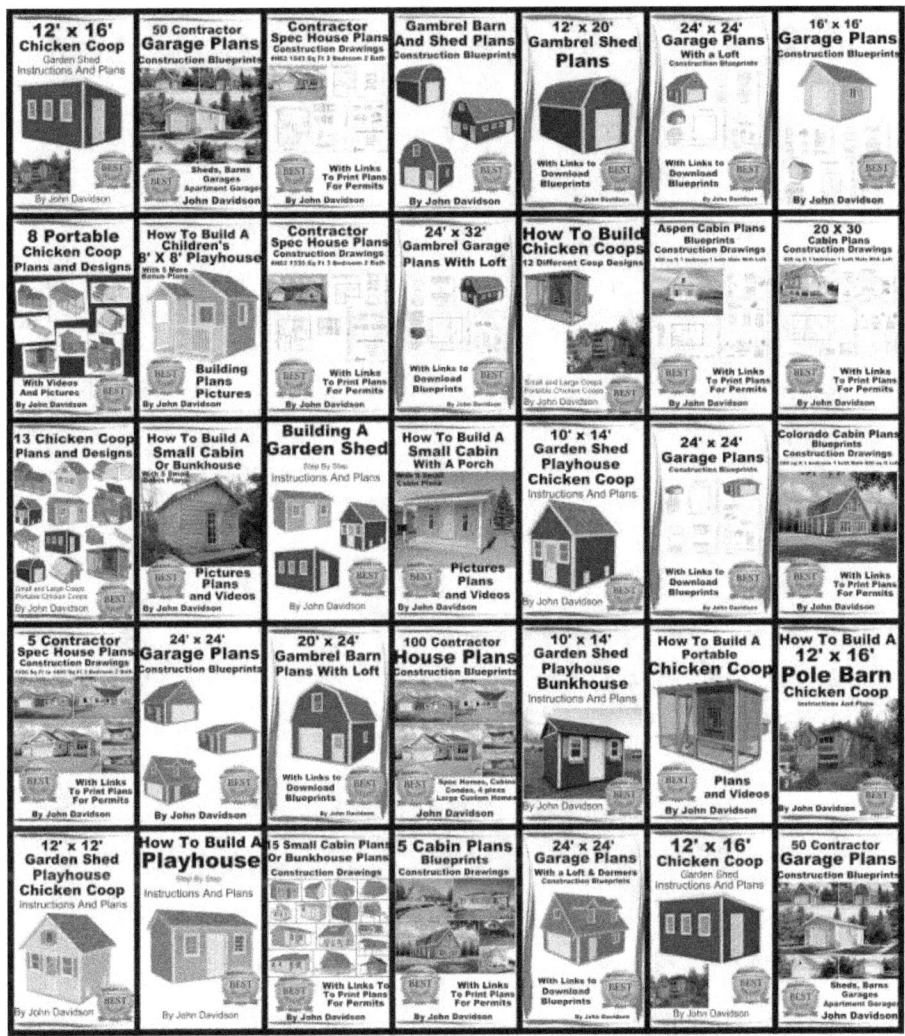

Entrepreneur Book Series

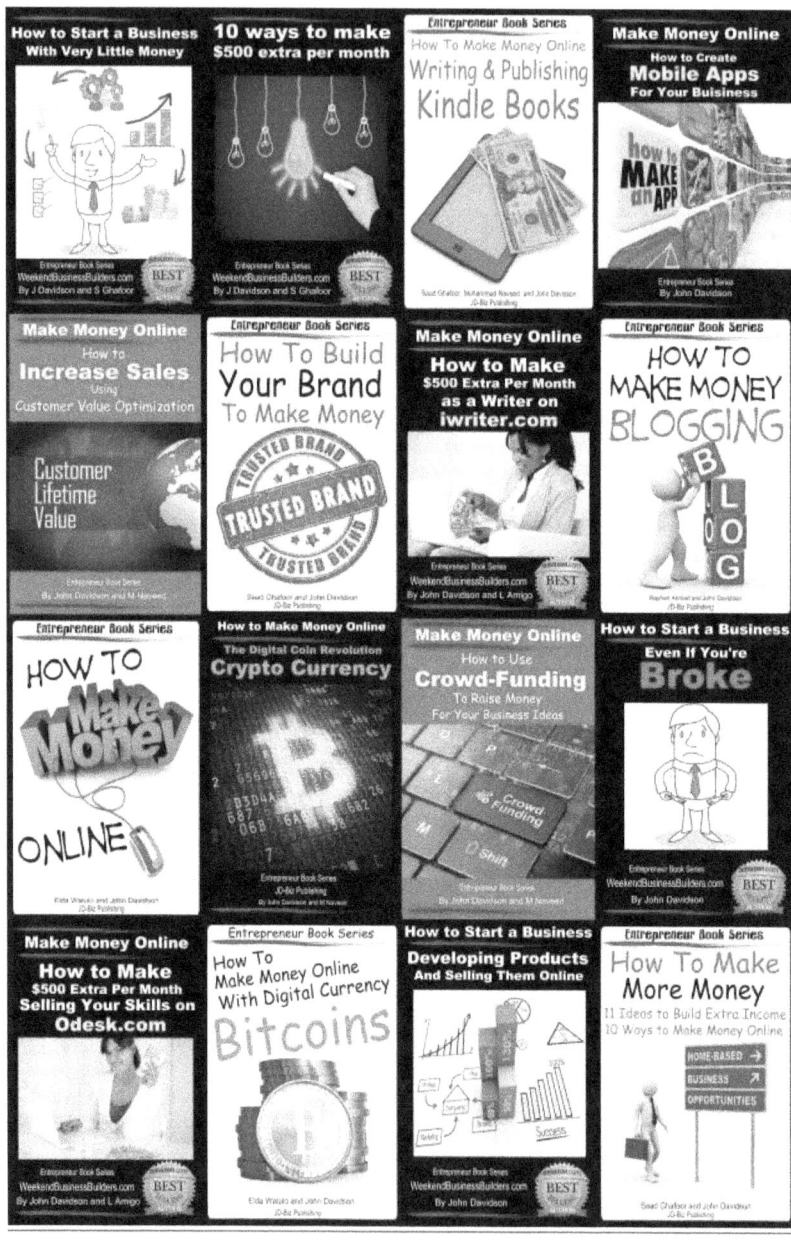

Our books are available at

1. Amazon.com

2. Barnes and Noble

3. Itunes

4. Kobo

5. Smashwords

6. Google Play Books

Publisher

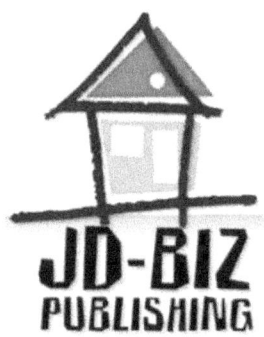

JD-Biz Corp

P O Box 374

Mendon, Utah 84325

http://www.jd-biz.com/

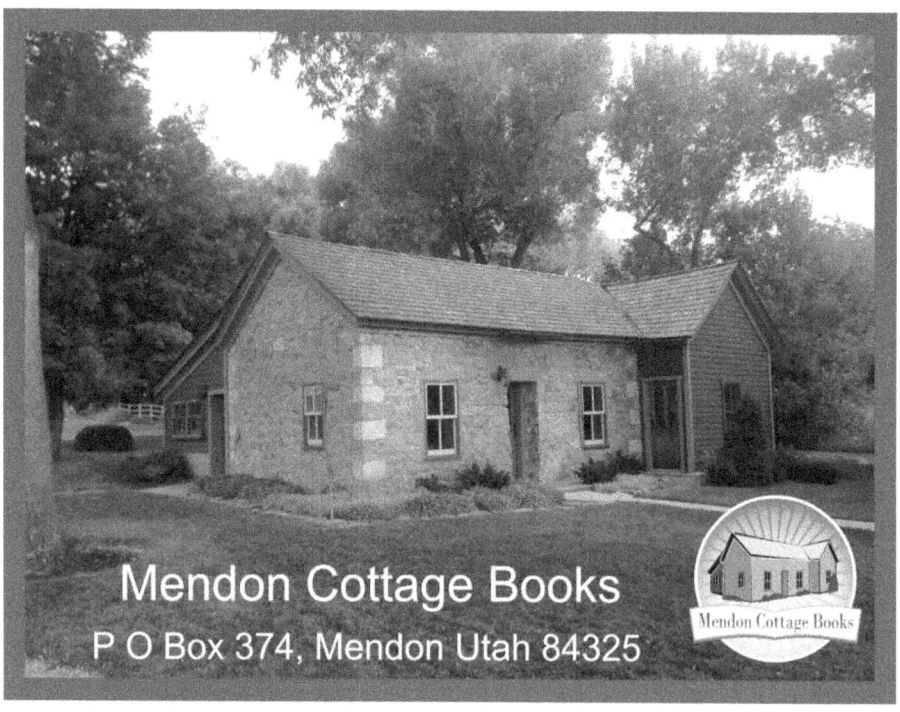

Mendon Cottage Books

P O Box 374, Mendon Utah 84325